OMAD COOKBOOK

MAIN COURSE - 60+ Breakfast, Lunch, Dinner and Dessert Recipes for intermittent fasting

TABLE OF CONTENTS

purposes solely, and is universal as so. The presentation of the information is without contract or any type of guarantee assurance.

The trademarks that are used are without any consent, and the publication of the trademark is without permission or backing by the trademark owner. All trademarks and brands within this book are for clarifying purposes only and are the owned by the owners themselves, not affiliated with this document.

Introduction

OMAD recipes for personal enjoyment but also for family enjoyment. You will love them for sure for how easy it is to prepare them.

BREAKFAST

BLUEBERRY PANCAKES

Serves: **4**

Prep Time: **10**   Minutes

Cook Time: **20**   Minutes

Total Time: **30**   Minutes

INGREDIENTS

- 1 cup whole wheat flour
- ¼ tsp baking soda
- ¼ tsp baking powder
- 1 cup blueberries
- 2 eggs
- 1 cup milk

DIRECTIONS

1. In a bowl combine all ingredients together and mix well
2. In a skillet heat olive oil

3. Pour ¼ of the batter and cook each pancake for 1-2 minutes per side

4. When ready remove from heat and serve

CHERRY PANCAKES

Serves: **4**

Prep Time: **10**   Minutes

Cook Time: **30**   Minutes

Total Time: **40**   Minutes

INGREDIENTS

- 1 cup whole wheat flour
- ¼ tsp baking soda
- ¼ tsp baking powder
- 1 cup cherries
- 2 eggs
- 1 cup milk

DIRECTIONS

1. In a bowl combine all ingredients together and mix well
2. In a skillet heat olive oil
3. Pour ¼ of the batter and cook each pancake for 1-2 minutes per side
4. When ready remove from heat and serve

BANANA PANCAKES

Serves: **4**

Prep Time: **10**   Minutes

Cook Time: **20**   Minutes

Total Time: **30**   Minutes

INGREDIENTS

- 1 cup whole wheat flour
- ¼ tsp baking soda
- ¼ tsp baking powder
- 1 cup mashed banana
- 2 eggs
- 1 cup milk

DIRECTIONS

1. In a bowl combine all ingredients together and mix well
2. In a skillet heat olive oil
3. Pour ¼ of the batter and cook each pancake for 1-2 minutes per side
4. When ready remove from heat and serve

LIME PANCAKES

Serves: **4**

Prep Time: **10** Minutes

Cook Time: **20** Minutes

Total Time: **30** Minutes

INGREDIENTS

- 1 cup whole wheat flour
- ¼ tsp baking soda
- ¼ tsp baking powder
- 1 cup lime
- 2 eggs
- 1 cup milk

DIRECTIONS

1. In a bowl combine all ingredients together and mix well
2. In a skillet heat olive oil
3. Pour ¼ of the batter and cook each pancake for 1-2 minutes per side
4. When ready remove from heat and serve

GUAVA PANCAKES

Serves: **4**

Prep Time: **10** Minutes

Cook Time: **30** Minutes

Total Time: **40** Minutes

INGREDIENTS

- 1 cup whole wheat flour
- ¼ tsp baking soda
- ¼ tsp baking powder
- 2 eggs
- 1 cup milk
- 1 cup guava

DIRECTIONS

1. In a bowl combine all ingredients together and mix well
2. In a skillet heat olive oil
3. Pour ¼ of the batter and cook each pancake for 1-2 minutes per side
4. When ready remove from heat and serve

APRICOT MUFFINS

Serves: **8-12**
Prep Time: **10**   Minutes

Cook Time: **20**   Minutes

Total Time: **30**   Minutes

INGREDIENTS

- 2 eggs
- 1 tablespoon olive oil
- 1 cup milk
- 2 cups whole wheat flour
- 1 tsp baking soda
- ¼ tsp baking soda
- 1 tsp ginger
- 1 cup apricot
- ¼ cup molasses

DIRECTIONS

1. In a bowl combine all dry ingredients
2. In another bowl combine all dry ingredients

3. Combine wet and dry ingredients together
4. Pour mixture into 8-12 prepared muffin cups, fill 2/3 of the cups
5. Bake for 18-20 minutes at 375 F
6. When ready remove from the oven and serve

PEACH MUFFINS

Serves:	*8-12*	
Prep Time:	*10*	Minutes
Cook Time:	*20*	Minutes
Total Time:	*30*	Minutes

INGREDIENTS

- 2 eggs
- 1 tablespoon olive oil
- 1 cup milk
- 2 cups whole wheat flour
- 1 tsp baking soda
- ¼ tsp baking soda
- 1 tsp cinnamon
- 1 cup mashed peaches

DIRECTIONS

1. In a bowl combine all dry ingredients
2. In another bowl combine all dry ingredients
3. Combine wet and dry ingredients together

4. Pour mixture into 8-12 prepared muffin cups, fill 2/3 of the cups

5. Bake for 18-20 minutes at 375 F

6. When ready remove from the oven and serve

Serves:	*8-12*	
Prep Time:	*10*	Minutes
Cook Time:	*20*	Minutes
Total Time:	*30*	Minutes

INGREDIENTS

- 2 eggs
- 1 tablespoon olive oil
- 1 cup milk
- 2 cups whole wheat flour
- 1 tsp baking soda
- ¼ tsp baking soda
- 1 tsp cinnamon
- 1 cup blueberries

DIRECTIONS

1. In a bowl combine all dry ingredients
2. In another bowl combine all dry ingredients
3. Combine wet and dry ingredients together

4. Fold in blueberries and mix well
5. Pour mixture into 8-12 prepared muffin cups, fill 2/3 of the cups
6. Bake for 18-20 minutes at 375 F
7. When ready remove from the oven and serve

PAPAYA MUFFINS

Serves: **8-12**

Prep Time: **10** Minutes

Cook Time: **20** Minutes

Total Time: **30** Minutes

INGREDIENTS

- 2 eggs
- 1 tablespoon olive oil
- 1 cup milk
- 2 cups whole wheat flour
- 1 tsp baking soda
- ¼ tsp baking soda
- 1 tsp cinnamon
- 1 cup papaya

DIRECTIONS

1. In a bowl combine all dry ingredients
2. In another bowl combine all dry ingredients
3. Combine wet and dry ingredients together

4. Pour mixture into 8-12 prepared muffin cups, fill 2/3 of the cups

5. Bake for 18-20 minutes at 375 F

6. When ready remove from the oven and serve

Serves: **8-12**
Prep Time: **10**   Minutes

Cook Time: **20**   Minutes

Total Time: **30**   Minutes

INGREDIENTS

- 2 eggs
- 1 tablespoon olive oil
- 1 cup milk
- 2 cups whole wheat flour
- 1 tsp baking soda
- ¼ tsp baking soda
- 1 tsp cinnamon
- 1 cup pineapple

DIRECTIONS

1. In a bowl combine all dry ingredients
2. In another bowl combine all dry ingredients
3. Combine wet and dry ingredients together

4. Pour mixture into 8-12 prepared muffin cups, fill 2/3 of the cups

5. Bake for 18-20 minutes at 375 F

6. When ready remove from the oven and serve

Serves:	*8-12*	
Prep Time:	*10*	Minutes
Cook Time:	*20*	Minutes
Total Time:	*30*	Minutes

INGREDIENTS

- 2 eggs
- 1 tablespoon olive oil
- 1 cup milk
- 2 cups whole wheat flour
- 1 tsp baking soda
- ¼ tsp baking soda
- 1 cup rhubarb

DIRECTIONS

1. In a bowl combine all dry ingredients
2. In another bowl combine all dry ingredients
3. Combine wet and dry ingredients together

4. Pour mixture into 8-12 prepared muffin cups, fill 2/3 of the cups

5. Bake for 18-20 minutes at 375 F

6. When ready remove from the oven and serve

Serves: **1**

Prep Time: **5**   Minutes

Cook Time: **10**   Minutes

Total Time: **15**   Minutes

INGREDIENTS

- 2 eggs
- ¼ tsp salt
- ¼ tsp black pepper
- 1 tablespoon olive oil
- ¼ cup cheese
- ¼ tsp basil
- 1 cup radish

DIRECTIONS

1. In a bowl combine all ingredients together and mix well
2. In a skillet heat olive oil and pour the egg mixture
3. Cook for 1-2 minutes per side

4. When ready remove omelette from the skillet and serve

Serves: *1*
Prep Time: *5*   Minutes

Cook Time: *10*   Minutes

Total Time: *15*   Minutes

INGREDIENTS

- **2 eggs**
- **¼ tsp salt**
- **¼ tsp black pepper**
- **1 tablespoon olive oil**
- **¼ cup cheese**
- **¼ tsp basil**
- **1 cup zucchini**

DIRECTIONS

1. **In a bowl combine all ingredients together and mix well**
2. **In a skillet heat olive oil and pour the egg mixture**
3. **Cook for 1-2 minutes per side**

4. When ready remove omelette from the skillet and serve

Serves: **1**

Prep Time: **5**   Minutes

Cook Time: **10** Minutes

Total Time: **15** Minutes

INGREDIENTS

- 2 eggs
- ¼ tsp salt
- ¼ tsp black pepper
- 1 tablespoon olive oil
- ¼ cup cheese
- ¼ tsp basil
- 1 cup corn

DIRECTIONS

1. In a bowl combine all ingredients together and mix well
2. In a skillet heat olive oil and pour the egg mixture
3. Cook for 1-2 minutes per side

4. When ready remove omelette from the skillet and serve

MUSHROOM OMELETTE

Serves: **1**

Prep Time: **5**   Minutes

Cook Time: **10**   Minutes

Total Time: **15**   Minutes

INGREDIENTS

- 2 eggs
- ¼ tsp salt
- ¼ tsp black pepper
- 1 tablespoon olive oil
- ¼ cup cheese
- ¼ tsp basil
- 1 cup mushrooms

DIRECTIONS

1. In a bowl combine all ingredients together and mix well
2. In a skillet heat olive oil and pour the egg mixture
3. Cook for 1-2 minutes per side

4. When ready remove omelette from the skillet and
   serve

Serves: **1**

Prep Time: **5**   Minutes

Cook Time: **10**   Minutes

Total Time: **15**   Minutes

INGREDIENTS

- 2 eggs
- ¼ tsp salt
- ¼ tsp black pepper
- 1 tablespoon olive oil
- ¼ cup cheese
- ¼ tsp basil
- 1 cup yams

DIRECTIONS

1. In a bowl combine all ingredients together and mix well
2. In a skillet heat olive oil and pour the egg mixture
3. Cook for 1-2 minutes per side

4. When ready remove omelette from the skillet and serve

BLUEBERRY OVERNIGHT OATS

Serves: **2**

Prep Time: **5** Minutes

Cook Time: **5** Minutes

Total Time: **10** Minutes

INGREDIENTS

- ½ cup oats
- ½ cup Greek yogurt
- 200 ml almond milk
- 1 cup peaches
- 1 cup blueberries

DIRECTIONS

1. In a bowl combine all ingredients together
2. Divide mixture into 2 jars and refrigerate
3. Serve in the morning

Serves: **2**
Prep Time: **5** Minutes

Cook Time: **10** Minutes

Total Time: **15** Minutes

INGREDIENTS

- 2 tortillas wraps
- 2 tablespoons peanut butter
- 1 banana
- 1 cup raspberries
- 1 cup blueberries
- 1 oz. almond flakes

DIRECTIONS

1. In a frying pan heat the wraps and spoon peanut butter on each tortilla wrap
2. Divide the fruits into the wraps and top with almond flakes
3. Serve when ready

Serves: **4**

Prep Time: **10**   Minutes

Cook Time: **20**   Minutes

Total Time: **30**   Minutes

INGREDIENTS

- 2 white potatoes
- 2 red peppers
- 1 red onion
- 1 tablespoon olive oil
- ¼ tsp cumin
- ¼ tsp cumin
- ½ lb. tomatoes
- 2 oz. spinach
- 2 eggs
- 1 avocado

DIRECTIONS

1. Place all the vegetables into a baking dish and drizzle olive oil

2. Scatter over the spices and toss to coat

3. Bake at 400 F for 18-20 minutes

4. While cooking crack the eggs over the vegetables and continue cooking until the vegetables are tender

5. When ready remove from the oven and serve

Serves: **6-8**
Prep Time: **10**   Minutes

Cook Time: **35**   Minutes

Total Time: **45**   Minutes

INGREDIENTS

- 2 bananas
- 2 eggs
- ¼ lb. dates
- 2 tablespoons Greek yogurt
- 1 tsp chia seeds
- 1 lb. self-rising flour
- 1 tsp coconut flakes
- ½ cup almond milk

DIRECTIONS

1. In a bowl combine all dry ingredients
2. In another bowl combine all wet ingredients

3. Fold wet ingredients into the dry mixture and mix well

4. Pour the dough into a loaf tin

5. Bake at 375 F for 30-35 minutes or until golden brown

6. When ready remove from the oven and serve

ALMOND PORRIDGE

Serves: **2**

Prep Time: **10** Minutes

Cook Time: **25** Minutes

Total Time: **35** Minutes

INGREDIENTS

- 5-6 plums
- 2-3 tablespoons maple syrup
- Orange from 1 orange
- ½ lb. oats
- ½ L almond milk
- 3-4 tablespoons almonds

DIRECTIONS

1. Place the plums on a baking tray and drizzle with maple syrup
2. Bake at 375 F for 20-25 minutes
3. In a saucepan add almond milk and remaining ingredients, bring to a boil
4. Cook on medium heat for 15-20 minutes

5. Divide the porridge between 2-3 bowls
6. Top with plums and serve

SIMPLE PIZZA RECIPE

Serves: **6-8**
Prep Time: **10** Minutes

Cook Time: **15** Minutes

Total Time: **25** Minutes

INGREDIENTS

- 1 pizza crust
- ½ cup tomato sauce
- ¼ black pepper
- 1 cup pepperoni slices
- 1 cup mozzarella cheese
- 1 cup olives

DIRECTIONS

1. Spread tomato sauce on the pizza crust
2. Place all the toppings on the pizza crust
3. Bake the pizza at 425 F for 12-15 minutes

4. When ready remove pizza from the oven and
   serve

ZUCCHINI PIZZA

Serves: **6-8**
Prep Time: **10**   Minutes

Cook Time: **15**   Minutes

Total Time: **25**   Minutes

INGREDIENTS

- 1 pizza crust
- ½ cup tomato sauce
- ¼ black pepper
- 1 cup zucchini slices
- 1 cup mozzarella cheese
- 1 cup olives

DIRECTIONS

1. Spread tomato sauce on the pizza crust
2. Place all the toppings on the pizza crust
3. Bake the pizza at 425 F for 12-15 minutes
4. When ready remove pizza from the oven and serve

Serves: **2**

Prep Time: **10** Minutes

Cook Time: **20** Minutes

Total Time: **30** Minutes

INGREDIENTS

- ½ lb. asparagus
- 1 tablespoon olive oil
- ½ red onion
- ¼ tsp salt
- 2 eggs
- 2 oz. cheddar cheese
- 1 garlic clove
- ¼ tsp dill

DIRECTIONS

1. In a bowl whisk eggs with salt and cheese
2. In a frying pan heat olive oil and pour egg mixture

3. Add remaining ingredients and mix well
4. Serve when ready

Serves: **2**
Prep Time: **10**   Minutes
Cook Time: **20**   Minutes
Total Time: **30**   Minutes

INGREDIENTS

- ½ lb. spinach
- 1 tablespoon olive oil
- ½ red onion
- ¼ tsp salt
- 2 eggs
- 2 oz. cheddar cheese
- 1 garlic clove
- ¼ tsp dill

DIRECTIONS

1. In a bowl whisk eggs with salt and cheese
2. In a frying pan heat olive oil and pour egg mixture

3. Add remaining ingredients and mix well
4. Serve when ready

CHEESE FRITATTA

Serves: **2**

Prep Time: **10**   Minutes

Cook Time: **20**   Minutes

Total Time: **30**   Minutes

INGREDIENTS

- 1 tablespoon olive oil
- ½ red onion
- ¼ tsp salt
- 2 eggs
- 1 cup cheddar cheese
- 1 garlic clove
- ¼ tsp dill

DIRECTIONS

1. In a bowl whisk eggs with salt and cheese
2. In a frying pan heat olive oil and pour egg mixture
3. Add remaining ingredients and mix well

4. Serve when ready

RHUBARB FRITATTA

Serves: **2**

Prep Time: **10**   Minutes

Cook Time: **20**   Minutes

Total Time: **30**   Minutes

INGREDIENTS

- 1 cup rhubarb
- 1 tablespoon olive oil
- ½ red onion
- ¼ tsp salt
- 2 oz. parmesan cheese
- 1 garlic clove
- ¼ tsp dill

DIRECTIONS

1. In a bowl whisk eggs with salt and parmesan cheese
2. In a frying pan heat olive oil and pour egg mixture
3. Add remaining ingredients and mix well

4. Serve when ready

Serves: **2**

Prep Time: **10** Minutes

Cook Time: **20** Minutes

Total Time: **30** Minutes

INGREDIENTS

- 1 cup broccoli
- 1 tablespoon olive oil
- ½ red onion
- 2 eggs
- ¼ tsp salt
- 2 oz. cheddar cheese
- 1 garlic clove
- ¼ tsp dill

DIRECTIONS

1. In a bowl whisk eggs with salt and cheese
2. In a frying pan heat olive oil and pour egg mixture

3. Add remaining ingredients and mix well
4. Serve when ready

TOMATO RISOTTO

Serves: **2**

Prep Time: **10** Minutes

Cook Time: **25** Minutes

Total Time: **35** Minutes

INGREDIENTS

- 2-3 tablespoons olive oil
- 1 red onion
- 1 lb. vine-ripened tomatoes
- 1 lb. risotto rice
- 1 cup vegetable stock
- 1 cup cheese
- 2 oz. basil

DIRECTIONS

1. In a pan heat olive oil and sauté onion until soft
2. Place the tomatoes on a baking tray, drizzle olive oil and roast at 350 F for 18-20 minutes
3. Add the rice, stock to the pan and cook until rice is tender

4. Add the cheese, basil, tomatoes and serve when
   ready

Serves: **2**

Prep Time: **10** Minutes

Cook Time: **50** Minutes

Total Time: **60** Minutes

INGREDIENTS

- 1 lb. butternut squash
- 3 tablespoons olive oil
- ¼ rolled pastry
- 2 eggs
- 200 ml double cream

DIRECTIONS

1. Roast the squash at 400 F for 18-20 minutes
2. Lay a baking paper on the pastry
3. Top with beans and bake for 12-15 minutes
4. Top the pastry with squash
5. Mix eggs, with double cream and pour over
6. Bake for another 20-25 minutes

7. When ready remove from the oven and serve

TOMATO TARTS

Serves: *2*
Prep Time: *10*   Minutes

Cook Time: *35*   Minutes

Total Time: *45*   Minutes

INGREDIENTS

- 1 lb. pastry
- 2-3 tsp tomato paste
- 1 lb. tomatoes
- 1 tablespoons olive oil
- 1 tablespoon capers
- 1 lb. broccoli

DIRECTIONS

1. Unroll the pastry sheet and cut into rectangles
2. Spread tomato paste over each tart and drizzle olive oil
3. Scatter over capers
4. Bake at 400 F for 18-20 minutes

5. Meanwhile boil the broccoli for 12-15 minutes or until tender

6. When ready remove from the oven and serve with cooked broccoli

TOMATO AND ONION PASTA

Serves: **2**

Prep Time: **10**   Minutes

Cook Time: **20**   Minutes

Total Time: **30**   Minutes

INGREDIENTS

- 1 tablespoon olive oil
- 1 onion
- ½ lb. penne pasta
- 2-3 garlic cloves
- 1 oz. parsley
- ½ lb. tomatoes
- ¼ lb. low fat sour cream

DIRECTIONS

1. Heat olive oil in a pan and sauté onion until soft
2. Add pasta, garlic, pasta and water to cover
3. Bring to a boil and simmer for 5-6 minutes
4. Add tomatoes and cook for another 4-5 minutes

5. Drain the pasta mixture and return to the pan
6. Stir in soured cream
7. Garnish with parsley and serve

TOFU SALAD

Serves: **1**

Prep Time: **5** Minutes

Cook Time: **5** Minutes

Total Time: **10** Minutes

INGREDIENTS

- 1 pack tofu
- 1 cup chopped vegetables (carrots, cucumber)

DRESSING

- 1 tablespoon sesame oil
- 1 tablespoon mustard
- 1 tablespoon brown rice vinegar
- 1 tablespoon soya sauce

DIRECTIONS

1. In a bowl combine all ingredients together
2. Add salad dressing, toss well and serve

Serves: *1*
Prep Time: 5   Minutes

Cook Time: 5   Minutes

Total Time: *10*   Minutes

INGREDIENTS

- 1 cup cooked couscous
- ¼ cup pine nuts
- 1 shallot
- 2 cloves garlic
- 1 can chickpeas
- 2 oz. low fat cheese
- 1 zucchini

DIRECTIONS

1. In a bowl combine all ingredients together
2. Add salad dressing, toss well and serve

BROCCOLI SALAD

Serves: **1**

Prep Time: **5**   Minutes

Cook Time: **5**   Minutes

Total Time: **10**   Minutes

INGREDIENTS

- 1 broccoli
- 1 cup tomatoes
- 1 cup feta cheese
- ½ cup almonds
- 1 cup lemon salad dressing

DIRECTIONS

1. In a bowl combine all ingredients together
2. Add salad dressing, toss well and serve

Serves: **1**
Prep Time: **5**   Minutes

Cook Time: **5**   Minutes

Total Time: **10**   Minutes

INGREDIENTS

- ½ cup sun-dried tomatoes
- ½ cup parmesan
- 1 tablespoon lemon juice
- 1 garlic clove
- ¼ cup olive oil
- 1 cup lemon salad dressing

DIRECTIONS

1. In a bowl combine all ingredients together
2. Add salad dressing, toss well and serve

CARROT-EDAMAME SALAD

Serves: **1**

Prep Time: **5**   Minutes

Cook Time: **5**   Minutes

Total Time: **10** Minutes

INGREDIENTS

- 4 oz. romaine lettuce
- 1 cup edamame
- 1 cup cabbage
- ¼ cup red onion
- 1 red bell pepper
- ¼ cup cilantro

DIRECTIONS

1. In a bowl combine all ingredients together
2. Add salad dressing, toss well and serve

CAULIFLOWER & FARRO SALAD

Serves: **1**

Prep Time: **5**   Minutes

Cook Time: **5**   Minutes

Total Time: **10** Minutes

INGREDIENTS

- 1 cauliflower
- 1 tablespoon olive oil
- ¼ tsp black pepper
- 1 cup cooked Farro
- 2 garlic cloves
- ¼ cup feta cheese
- 1 avocado

DIRECTIONS

1. In a bowl combine all ingredients together
2. Add salad dressing, toss well and serve

ARUGULA &CHICKPEA SALAD

Serves: **1**

Prep Time: **5** Minutes

Cook Time: **5** Minutes

Total Time: **10** Minutes

INGREDIENTS

- 1 cup cooked chickpeas
- 2 carrots
- ¼ cup feta cheese
- 4 cups arugula
- 1 cup lemon salad dressing

DIRECTIONS

1. In a bowl combine all ingredients together
2. Add salad dressing, toss well and serve

Serves: *1*
Prep Time: *5*   Minutes

Cook Time: *5*   Minutes

Total Time: *10*   Minutes

INGREDIENTS

- 2 cups romaine lettuce
- 1 head radicchio
- 1 red onion
- 1 cup cherry tomatoes
- ¼ cup sun-dried tomatoes
- 1 can cooked chickpeas
- 1 cup Italian vinaigrette

DIRECTIONS

1. In a bowl combine all ingredients together
2. Add salad dressing, toss well and serve

CARROTS & DILL SALAD

Serves: *1*
Prep Time: *5*   Minutes
Cook Time: *5*   Minutes
Total Time: *10*   Minutes

INGREDIENTS

- 1 cup cooked chickpeas
- 1 cup carrots
- ½ cup celery
- ¼ cup dill
- ¼ cup olive oil
- 1 garlic clove

DIRECTIONS

1. In a bowl combine all ingredients together
2. Add salad dressing, toss well and serve

Serves: **1**
Prep Time: **5** Minutes

Cook Time: **5** Minutes

Total Time: **10** Minutes

INGREDIENTS

- 1 cup cooked quinoa
- ½ cup cooked chickpeas
- 1 cup baby spinach
- ½ cup greens
- ½ cup feta cheese
- ½ cup tomatoes

DIRECTIONS

1. In a bowl combine all ingredients together
2. Add salad dressing, toss well and serve

DINNER

CAULIFLOWER RECIPE

Serves: **6-8**

Prep Time: **10** Minutes

Cook Time: **15** Minutes

Total Time: **25** Minutes

INGREDIENTS

- 1 pizza crust
- ½ cup tomato sauce
- ¼ black pepper
- 1 cup cauliflower
- 1 cup mozzarella cheese
- 1 cup olives

DIRECTIONS

1. Spread tomato sauce on the pizza crust
2. Place all the toppings on the pizza crust
3. Bake the pizza at 425 F for 12-15 minutes

4. When ready remove pizza from the oven and serve

Serves: **6-8**

Prep Time: **10**   Minutes

Cook Time: **15**   Minutes

Total Time: **25**   Minutes

INGREDIENTS

- 1 pizza crust
- ½ cup tomato sauce
- ¼ black pepper
- 1 cup broccoli
- 1 cup mozzarella cheese
- 1 cup olives

DIRECTIONS

1. Spread tomato sauce on the pizza crust
2. Place all the toppings on the pizza crust
3. Bake the pizza at 425 F for 12-15 minutes
4. When ready remove pizza from the oven and serve

TOMATOES & HAM PIZZA

Serves: **6-8**

Prep Time: **10**   Minutes

Cook Time: **15**   Minutes

Total Time: **25**   Minutes

INGREDIENTS

- 1 pizza crust
- ½ cup tomato sauce
- ¼ black pepper
- 1 cup pepperoni slices
- 1 cup tomatoes
- 6-8 ham slices
- 1 cup mozzarella cheese
- 1 cup olives

DIRECTIONS

1. Spread tomato sauce on the pizza crust
2. Place all the toppings on the pizza crust
3. Bake the pizza at 425 F for 12-15 minutes

4. When ready remove pizza from the oven and serve

TARO SOUP

Serves: **4**

Prep Time: **10**   Minutes

Cook Time: **20**   Minutes

Total Time: **30**   Minutes

INGREDIENTS

- 1 tablespoon olive oil
- ¼ red onion
- ½ cup all-purpose flour
- ¼ tsp salt
- ¼ tsp pepper
- 1 can vegetable broth
- 1 cup heavy cream
- 1 cup taro

DIRECTIONS

1. In a saucepan heat olive oil and sauté onion until tender
2. Add remaining ingredients to the saucepan and bring to a boil

3. When all the vegetables are tender transfer to a blender and blend until smooth

4. Pour soup into bowls, garnish with parsley and serve

Serves: **4**

Prep Time: **10**   Minutes

Cook Time: **20**   Minutes

Total Time: **30**   Minutes

INGREDIENTS

- 1 tablespoon olive oil
- 1 lb. tomato
- ¼ red onion
- ½ cup all-purpose flour
- ¼ tsp salt
- ¼ tsp pepper
- 1 can vegetable broth
- 1 cup heavy cream

DIRECTIONS

1. In a saucepan heat olive oil and sauté onion until tender
2. Add remaining ingredients to the saucepan and bring to a boil

3. When all the vegetables are tender transfer to a blender and blend until smooth

4. Pour soup into bowls, garnish with parsley and serve

SPINACH SOUP

Serves: **4**

Prep Time: **10**   Minutes

Cook Time: **20**   Minutes

Total Time: **30**   Minutes

INGREDIENTS

- 1 tablespoon olive oil
- 1 lb. spinach
- ¼ red onion
- ½ cup all-purpose flour
- ¼ tsp salt
- ¼ tsp pepper
- 1 can vegetable broth
- 1 cup heavy cream

DIRECTIONS

1. In a saucepan heat olive oil and sauté spinach until tender
2. Add remaining ingredients to the saucepan and bring to a boil

3. When all the vegetables are tender transfer to a blender and blend until smooth

4. Pour soup into bowls, garnish with parsley and serve

SPINACH SOUP

Serves: **4**

Prep Time: **10**   Minutes

Cook Time: **20**   Minutes

Total Time: **30**   Minutes

INGREDIENTS

- 1 tablespoon olive oil
- 1 lb. spinach
- ¼ red onion
- ½ cup all-purpose flour
- ¼ tsp salt
- ¼ tsp pepper
- 1 can vegetable broth
- 1 cup heavy cream

DIRECTIONS

1. In a saucepan heat olive oil and sauté onion until tender
2. Add remaining ingredients to the saucepan and bring to a boil

3. When all the vegetables are tender transfer to a blender and blend until smooth

4. Pour soup into bowls, garnish with parsley and serve

POTATO SOUP

Serves: **4**

Prep Time: **10**   Minutes

Cook Time: **20**   Minutes

Total Time: **30**   Minutes

INGREDIENTS

- 1 tablespoon olive oil
- 1 lb. mushrooms
- ¼ red onion
- ½ cup all-purpose flour
- ¼ tsp salt
- ¼ tsp pepper
- 1 can vegetable broth
- 1 cup heavy cream

DIRECTIONS

1. In a saucepan heat olive oil and sauté potatoes until tender
2. Add remaining ingredients to the saucepan and bring to a boil

3. When all the vegetables are tender transfer to a blender and blend until smooth

4. Pour soup into bowls, garnish with parsley and serve

MACA SMOOTHIE

Serves: **1**

Prep Time: **5** Minutes

Cook Time: **5** Minutes

Total Time: **10** Minutes

INGREDIENTS

- 2 cups hemp milk
- 1 cup ice
- ¼ cup lemon juice
- 2 mangoes
- 1 tablespoon flaxseeds
- 1 tsp maca power
- 1 tsp vanilla extract

DIRECTIONS

1. In a blender place all ingredients and blend until smooth
2. Pour smoothie in a glass and serve

MACA SMOOTHIE

Serves: **1**
Prep Time: **5**   Minutes
Cook Time: **5**   Minutes
Total Time: **10** Minutes

INGREDIENTS

- 2 cups hemp milk
- 1 cup ice
- ¼ cup lemon juice
- 2 mangoes
- 1 tablespoon flaxseeds
- 1 tsp maca power
- 1 tsp vanilla extract

DIRECTIONS

1. In a blender place all ingredients and blend until smooth
2. Pour smoothie in a glass and serve

BABY SPINACH SMOOTHIE

Serves: *1*
Prep Time: *5*   Minutes

Cook Time: *5*   Minutes

Total Time: *10*   Minutes

INGREDIENTS

- 1 cup cherry juice
- 1 cup spinach
- 1 cup vanilla yoghurt
- 1 avocado
- 1 cup berries
- 1 tablespoon chia seeds

DIRECTIONS

1. In a blender place all ingredients and blend until smooth
2. Pour smoothie in a glass and serve

SUNRISE SMOOTHIE

Serves: *1*
Prep Time: *5*   Minutes

Cook Time: *5*   Minutes

Total Time: *10* Minutes

INGREDIENTS

- 1 cup coconut milk
- 1 banana
- ¼ cup lemon juice
- ¼ mango
- 1 tsp almonds
- 1 cup ice

DIRECTIONS

1. In a blender place all ingredients and blend until smooth
2. Pour smoothie in a glass and serve

CUCUMBER SMOOTHIE

Serves: **1**

Prep Time: **5** Minutes

Cook Time: **5** Minutes

Total Time: **10** Minutes

INGREDIENTS

- 1 cup vanilla yoghurt
- 1 cup cucumber
- 2 tablespoons dill
- 1 tablespoon basil
- 2 tablespoons mint
- 1 cup ice

DIRECTIONS

1. In a blender place all ingredients and blend until smooth
2. Pour smoothie in a glass and serve

CHERRY SMOOTHIE

Serves: **1**

Prep Time: **5**   Minutes

Cook Time: **5**   Minutes

Total Time: **10** Minutes

INGREDIENTS

- 1 can cherries
- 2 tablespoons peanut butter
- 1 tablespoon honey
- 1 cup Greek Yoghurt
- 1 cup coconut milk

DIRECTIONS

1. In a blender place all ingredients and blend until smooth
2. Pour smoothie in a glass and serve

Serves: *1*
Prep Time: **5** Minutes

Cook Time: **5** Minutes

Total Time: *10* Minutes

INGREDIENTS

- 2 bananas
- 1 cup Greek Yoghurt
- 1 tablespoon honey
- 1 tablespoon cocoa powder
- ½ cup chocolate chips
- ¼ cup almond milk

DIRECTIONS

1. In a blender place all ingredients and blend until smooth
2. Pour smoothie in a glass and serve

TOFU SMOOTHIE

Serves: **1**

Prep Time: **5** Minutes

Cook Time: **5** Minutes

Total Time: **10** Minutes

INGREDIENTS

- 1 cup blueberries
- ¼ cup tofu
- ¼ cup pomegranate juice
- 1 cup ice
- ½ cup agave nectar

DIRECTIONS

1. In a blender place all ingredients and blend until smooth
2. Pour smoothie in a glass and serve

COCONUT SMOOTHIE

Serves: **1**

Prep Time: **5**   Minutes

Cook Time: **5**   Minutes

Total Time: **10**   Minutes

INGREDIENTS

- 1 cup blueberries
- 2 bananas
- 1 cup coconut flakes
- 1 cup coconut milk
- ¼ tsp vanilla essence

DIRECTIONS

1. In a blender place all ingredients and blend until smooth
2. Pour smoothie in a glass and serve

BERRY-BANANA SMOOTHIE

Serves: **1**

Prep Time: **5** Minutes

Cook Time: **5** Minutes

Total Time: **10** Minutes

INGREDIENTS

- 1 banana
- 1 cup blueberries
- 1 cup vanilla yogurt
- ¼ tablespoon cinnamon
- 1 cup berries

DIRECTIONS

1. In a blender place all ingredients and blend until smooth
2. Pour smoothie in a glass and serve

Serves: *1*
Prep Time: *5*   Minutes

Cook Time: *5*   Minutes

Total Time: *10*   Minutes

INGREDIENTS

- 2 mangoes
- 1 tablespoon honey
- 1 cup yogurt
- 2 kiwis
- 1 cup ice
- 1 cup spinach
- ¼ tsp mint

DIRECTIONS

1. In a blender place all ingredients and blend until smooth
2. Pour smoothie in a glass and serve

THANK YOU FOR READING THIS BOOK!

Made in the USA
San Bernardino, CA
12 February 2020